Contents

Written by E Mark Pelmore

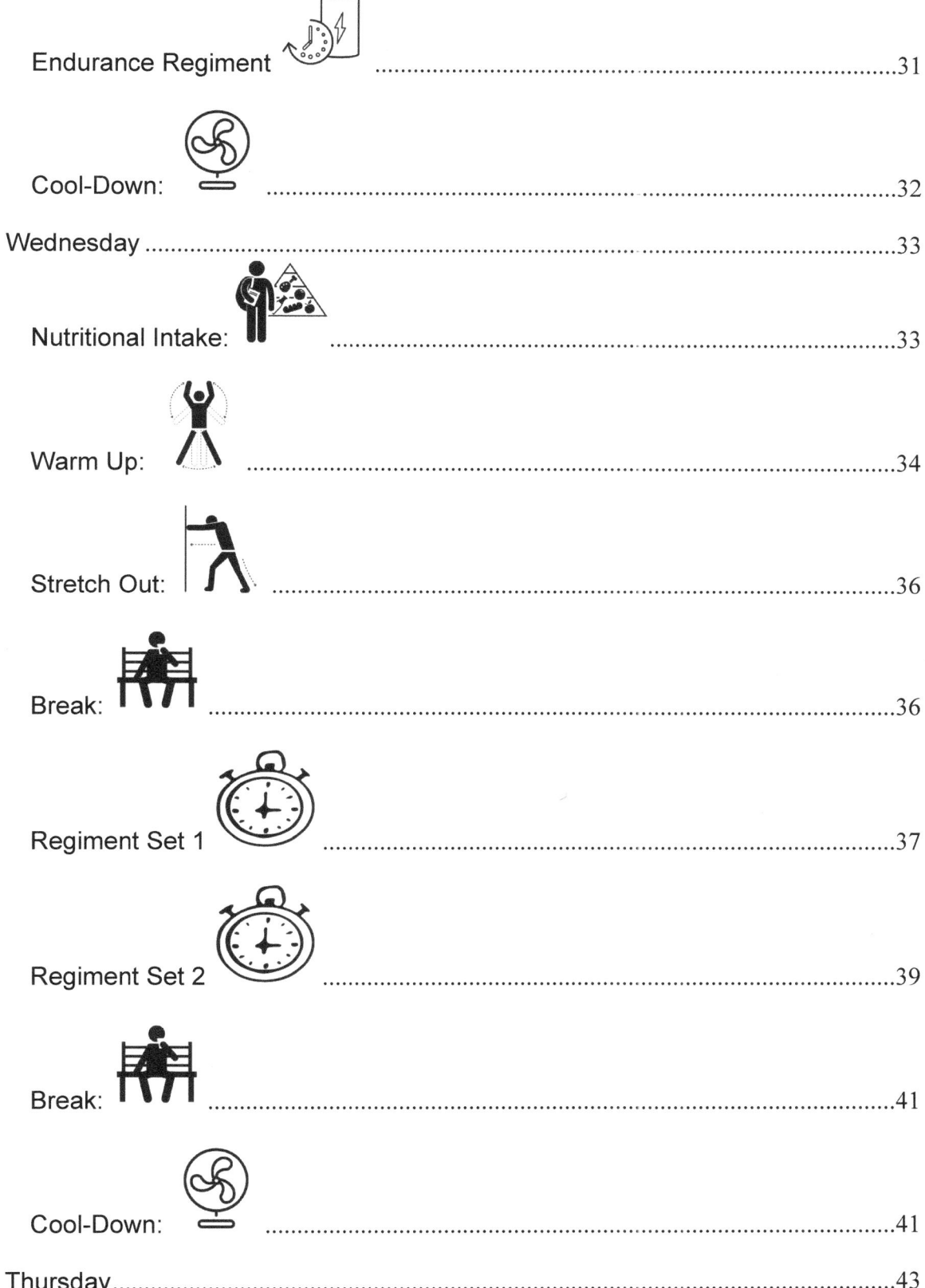
Written by E Mark Pelmore

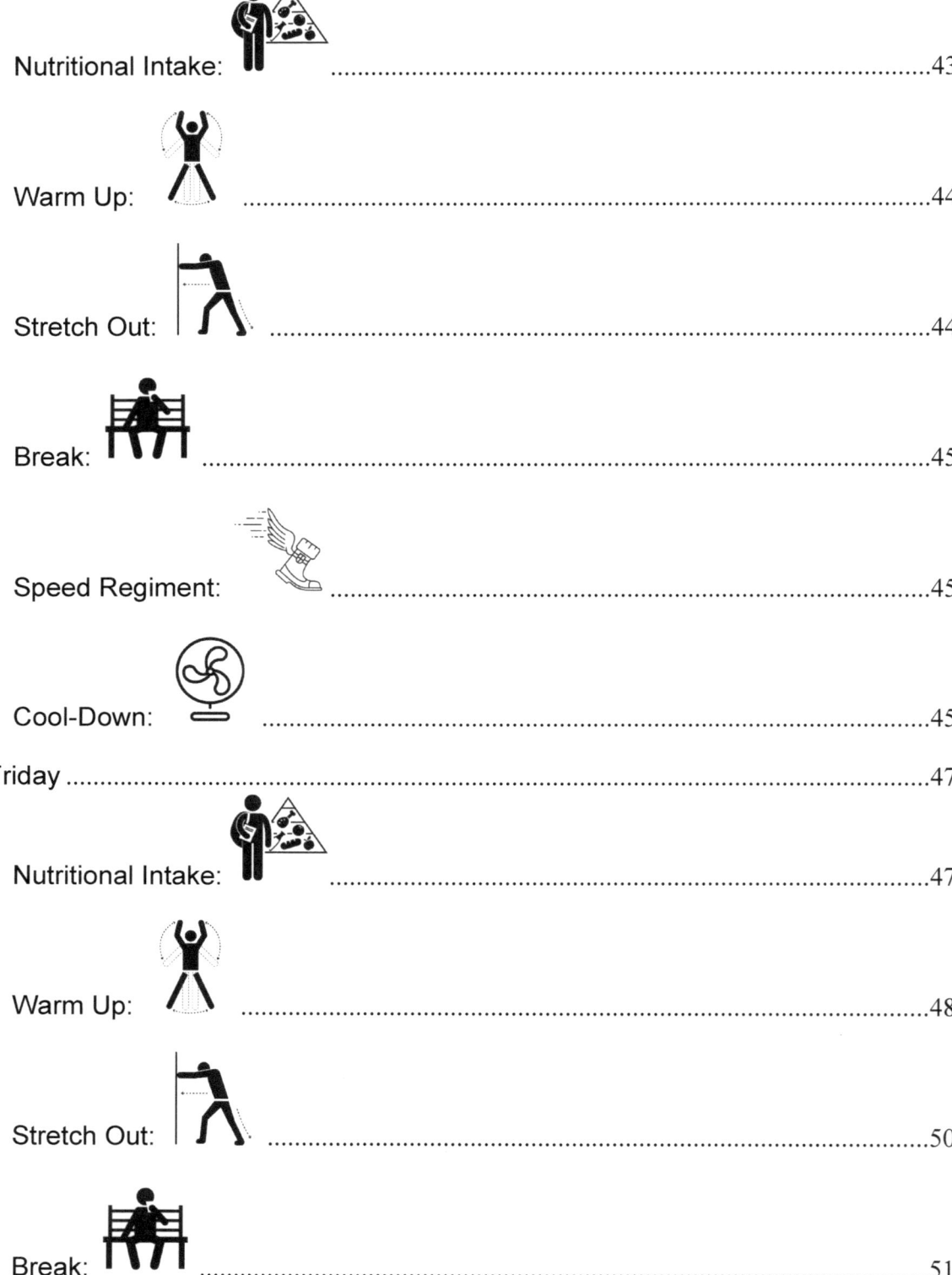

Written by E Mark Pelmore

Dedication:

Thank you, to my Lord and Savior, for giving me the desire and skill-set to accomplish something to help guide others.

Thank you to my Wife, (Crystal Danyel), for the love, patience, and understanding while I spent a great amount of time and effort developing the content of this Regiment.

Thank you to the US Army for developing the physical training knowledge & practices to design the Pulsate Regiment ©.

Thank you to the Lincoln & Hill, for seeing this Regiment as a viable asset to the mission & vision to combat obesity in the people you have direct contact with.

Tags & Legend

Alternate Tag: depicts a substitute activity for Cardio related exercises of the Regiment

Break Tag: depicts a stoppage in exercise for a designated time of the Regiment

Cardio Tag: depicts a heart rate related exercise of the Regiment

Cool-Down Tag: depicts the winding down exercises of the Regiment

Dance Experience Tag: depicts a dancing style Cardio exercise of the Regiment

Distance Tag: depicts a designated distance to run in and Speed or Endurance related exercise of the Regiment

Drink Water Tag: depicts required consumption of water throughout the deployment of the Regiment

Endurance Tag: depicts an Endurance related exercise of the Regiment

Food Intake Tag: depicts the tracking of food consumed in a 24 interval

Monitor Tag: depicts a need to monitor vitals during deployment of the Regiment

Muscular System Tag: depicts something related to the Muscle Groups

Nutritional Intake Tag: depicts the recommended calorie intake for age and gender in 24-hour intervals

Pace Tag: depicts the designated activity or movement rate for an exercise of the Regiment

Physician Tag: depicts the seeking of medical attention

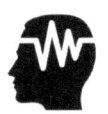 Pilates Tag: depicts a stretching style Cardio exercise of the Regiment

Pulsate Tag: depicts activity within the completion of the Regiment

Pulsate Regiment Tag: depicts the Pulsate Regiment Brand ©

Regiment Set Tag: depicts a designated number of intervals to complete the Regiment

Rest Tag: depicts required recharging of body throughout the deployment of the Regiment

Speed Tag: depicts an Speed related exercise of the Regiment

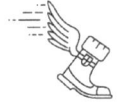 Stationary Machine Tag: depicts a dancing style Cardio exercise of the Regiment

Stretch-Out Tag: depicts the transitions from Warm Up to executing exercises of the Regiment

Track Tag: depicts the designated location and distance of a Speed or Endurance related exercise of the Regiment

Written by E Mark Pelmore

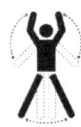 Warm-Up Tag: depicts the initiating exercises of the Regiment

 Water Aerobics Tag: depicts a water style Cardio exercise of the Regiment

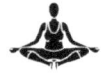 Wind Resistant Tag: depicts a personal accessory for resistance training in exercise of the Regiment

 Yoga Tag: depicts a balancing style Cardio exercise of the Regiment

Zumba Tag: depicts a group dancing style Cardio exercise of the Regiment

Pulsate the Regiment ©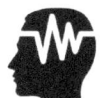

Pulsate the Regiment is designed as a high intensity interval training (HIIT) but structure to develop individual trainee to increase their ability to increase their participation.

HIIT

We choose the HIIT format because it doesn't require equipment or a great amount of time or space. In our regiment the short bursts are to help build intensity and capability. The purpose behind the regiment was a create a way to for everyone to understand their body and find a way to help heal or reshape their bodies is suffering from a myriad of symptoms. To help those that don't understand their body's, we provide a brief synopsis of the three main types, but each person is designed uniquely.

Somatotypes

There are three general types of bodies known as somatotypes, characteristics of two or even three of the categories is possible.

Ectomorphs

This body type is lean. This body type is typically low in body fat and has difficulty gaining weight. Today it is promoted as Ectomorphs are the desirable body types, but it is not always health risk free for some individuals.

Endomorphs

This body type is a combination of muscle and fat. This body type is at a higher risk of obesity and other serious health consequences. Individuals with Endomorphic body structures can survive normal sickness and injuries better, with factors like bone density.

Mesomorphs

This body type is both lean & muscular. This body type often fluctuates in weight without strenuous effort.

The regiment was designed with the body types in min to maximize the individual's potential without creating extra health risk in the process.

Major Muscle Groups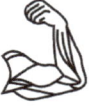

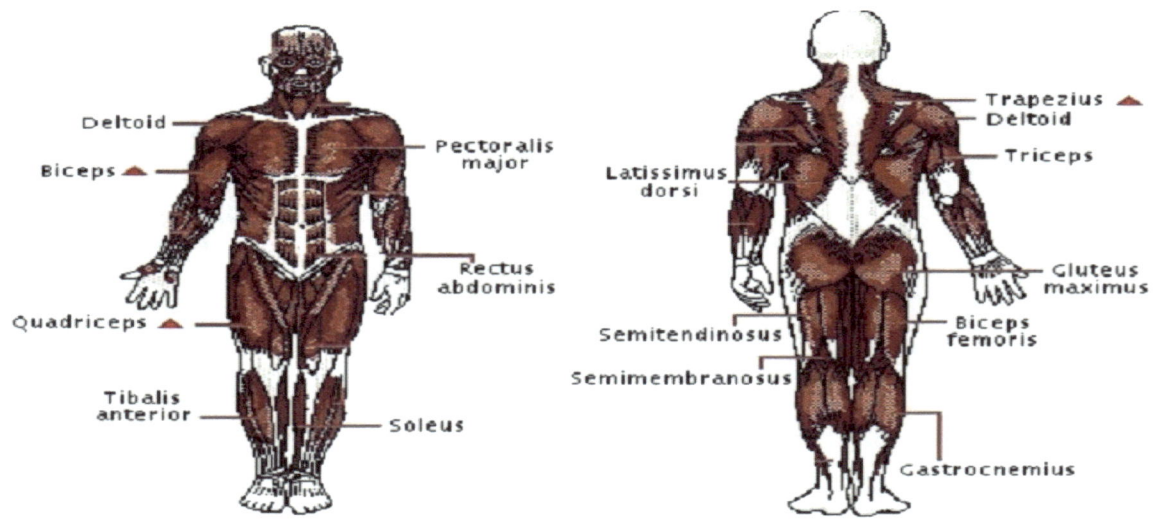

Your skeletal muscular system is made up of approximately 650 layers connected to your bones (often quoted as the number of muscle in body). The muscular system is broken into major muscle groupings.

Muscle Group	Location	Function	Strengthen
Abdominal	Stomach	Postural Alignment	Crunches or variation
Biceps	Upper Arm FR	Lifting or Pulling	Curls or variation
Deltoids	TP Shoulder	Overhead Lifting	Push Ups, Bench, Arm Raises
Erector Spinae	Lower BK	Postural Alignment	Core Extensions
Gastrocnemius & Soleus	Lower Leg BK	Push Off	Calf Raises
Gluteus	Buttocks	Climbing, Walking	Squats, Leg Press
Hamstring	Thigh BK	Climbing, Walking	Squats, Lunges Leg Extension & Curls
Latissimus Dorsi	Mid BK	Postural Alignment,	Pull Ups, Chin Ups, Pull Downs
Rhomboids	BW Shoulder Blades	Pulling	Chin Ups, Bent Arm Rows
Oblique's	Side	Rotation & Flexion	Twisting Crunches
Pectoralis	Upper Chest	Pushing	Push Ups, Pull Ups, Bench
Quadriceps	Thigh FR	Climbing, Walking	Squats, Lunges, Leg Presses
Trapezius	Upper & Mid BK	Moves Head Sideways	Shoulder Shrugs, Upright Rows
Triceps	Upper Arm BK	Pushing	Dips, Push Ups

Before moving forward into physical exercise or training make sure you have consulted with your physician to participate in the following activities.

Written by E Mark Pelmore

Being prepared physically also requires looking into your current diet plan or nutritional intake to better compliment you becoming active. Whether you're at those beginning levels, maintaining your current level of activity or ramping up to that next level of training a complimentary dietary plan is critical.

Disclaimer: ONLY attempt what you are capable of doing throughout the entire training regimen at the pace level you're currently at.

Reminders:

An appropriate complimentary diet regiment 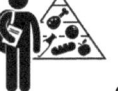 **& eating habits**

maximizes the Regiment. If you have a medical condition, please seek the

advice of your physician or other qualified health provider before attempting these rigorous exercises.

Sunday

Nutritional Intake: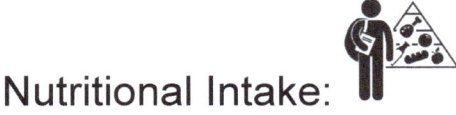

Age and gender	Estimated calories for those who do NO physically active	
	Total daily calorie needs*	Daily limit for empty calories
Girls 10-13 yrs.	1600 calories	120
Boys 10-13 yrs.	1800 calories	160
Girls 14-18 yrs.	1800 calories	160
Boys 14-18 yrs.	2200 calories	265
Females 19-30 yrs.	2000 calories	260
Males 19-30 yrs.	2400 calories	330
Females 31-50 yrs.	1800 calories	160
Males 31-50 yrs.	2200 calories	265
Females 51+ yrs.	1600 calories	120
Males 51+ yrs.	2000 calories	260

Track your Intake

Breakfast	Snack	Lunch	Snack	Dinner

Written by E Mark Pelmore

Rest the Body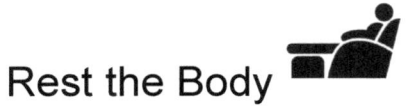

Rest the Body * – while replenishing the Mind & Soul

*drink plenty of water today, continuing that activity throughout the entire week;

*stretch muscles as needed on rest day & throughout the entire week;

Monday

Nutritional Intake: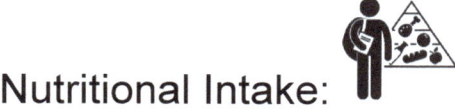

Age and gender	Estimated calories for those who do NO physically active	
	Total daily calorie needs*	Daily limit for empty calories
Girls 10-13 yrs.	1600 calories	120
Boys 10-13 yrs.	1800 calories	160
Girls 14-18 yrs.	1800 calories	160
Boys 14-18 yrs.	2200 calories	265
Females 19-30 yrs.	2000 calories	260
Males 19-30 yrs.	2400 calories	330
Females 31-50 yrs.	1800 calories	160
Males 31-50 yrs.	2200 calories	265
Females 51+ yrs.	1600 calories	120
Males 51+ yrs.	2000 calories	260

Track your Intake

Breakfast	Snack	Lunch	Snack	Dinner

Written by E Mark Pelmore

Warm Up: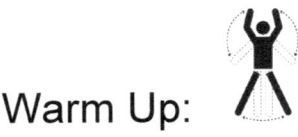

go through warm up regiment for Monday (each exercise 1 time for 20 seconds) at a light pace focusing on activating muscles and increasing heart rate

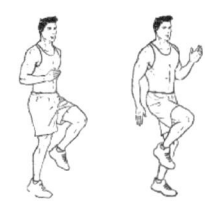

Jog in place (20 seconds)

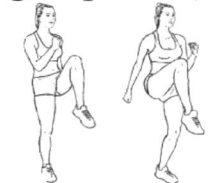

High Knees (20 seconds)

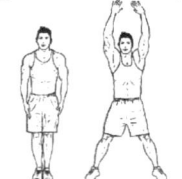

Power Jacks (20 seconds)

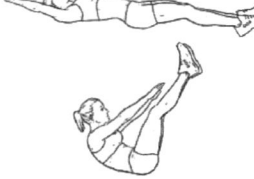

V Ups (20 seconds)

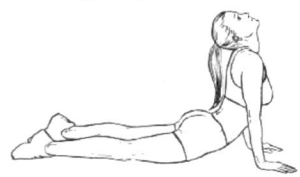

Back Extensions (20 seconds)

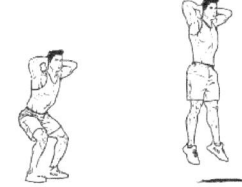

Squat Jumps (20 seconds)

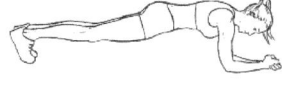

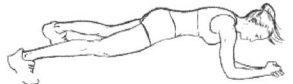

Plank Jacks (20 seconds)

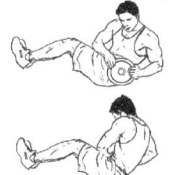

Oblique Twist (20 seconds)

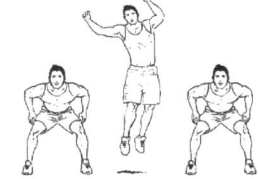

$(4 = 1 \sim \leftarrow \downarrow \rightarrow \uparrow)$

Globe Jumps (20 seconds)

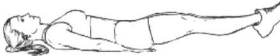

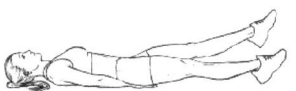

Flutter Kicks (20 seconds)

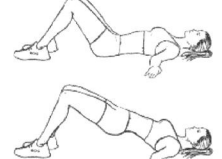

Bridge Ups (20 seconds)

Written by E Mark Pelmore

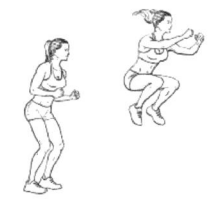

Jumping Power Knees (20 seconds)

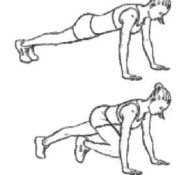

Mountain Climbers (20 seconds)

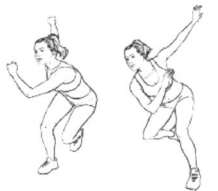

Skaters (20 seconds)

Stretch Out: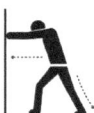

go through stretching regiment for Monday, focusing on elongating muscles

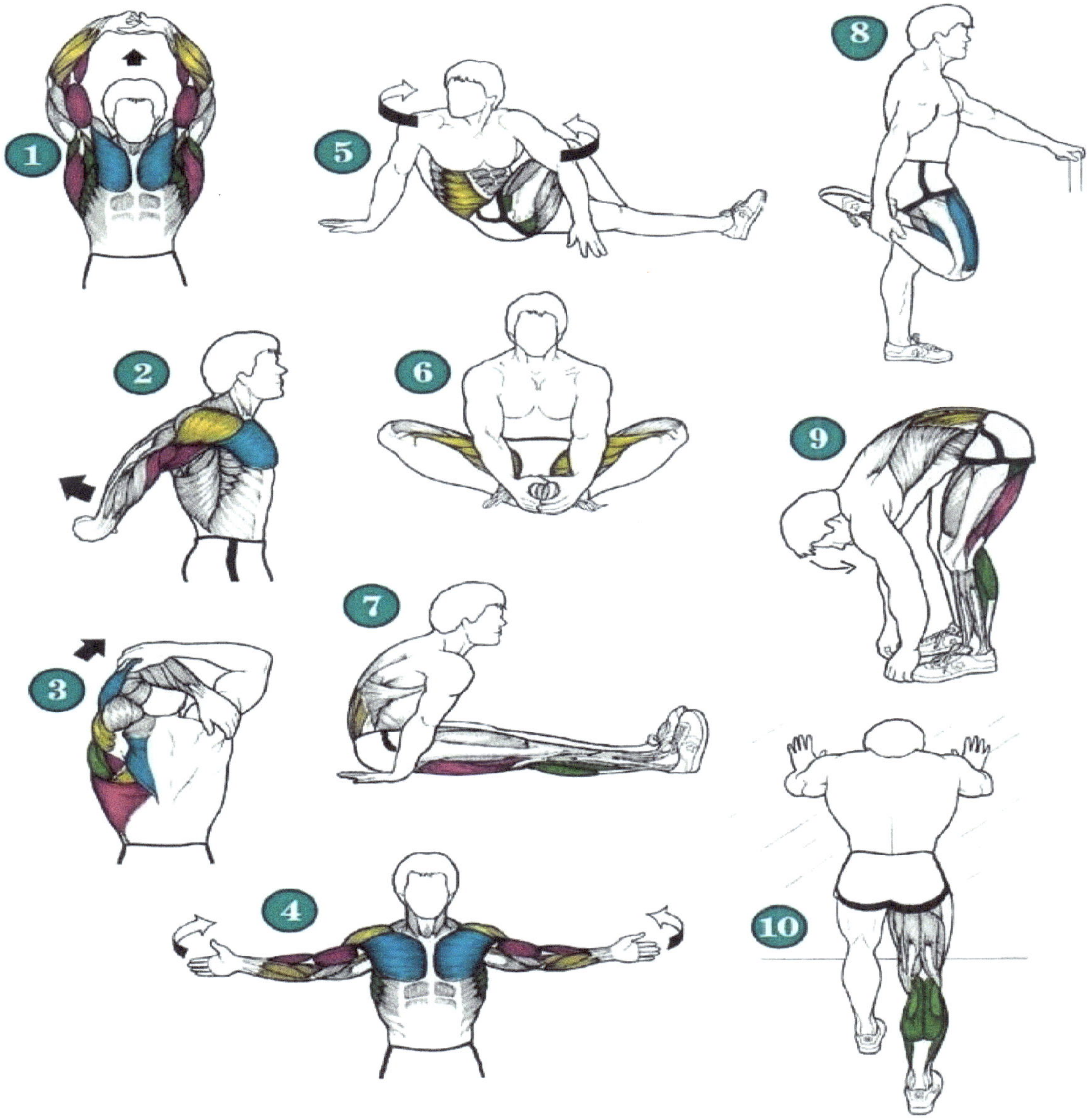

1

2

3

4

5

6

7

8

9

10

Break: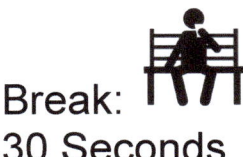
30 Seconds

Written by E Mark Pelmore

Pulsate:

go through regiment plan, first set (1) time for 30 seconds (each exercise 1 time for 30 seconds) at high intensity pace focusing on reaching target heart rate

Regiment Set 1

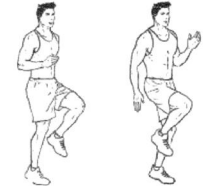

Jog in place (30 seconds)

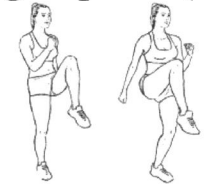

High Knees (30 seconds)

Power Jacks (30 seconds)

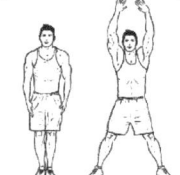

V Ups (30 seconds)

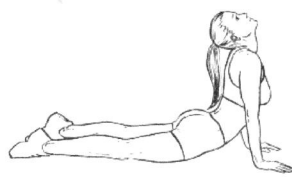

Back Extensions (30 seconds)

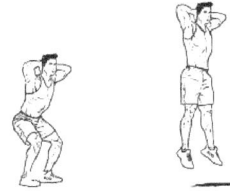

Squat Jumps (30 seconds)

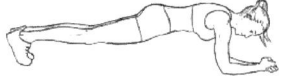

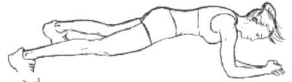

Plank Jacks (30 seconds)

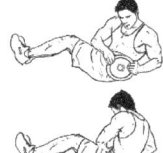

Oblique Twist (30 seconds)

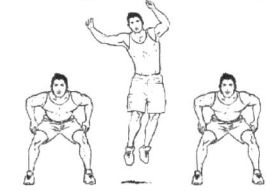

(4 = 1 ~ ←↓ →↑)

Globe Jumps (30 seconds)

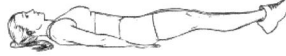

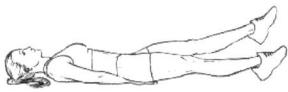

Flutter Kicks (30 seconds)

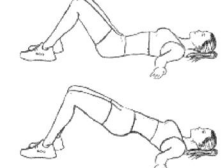

Bridge Ups (30 seconds)

Written by E Mark Pelmore

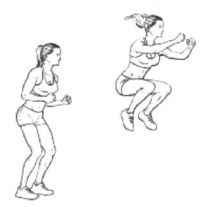

Jumping Power Knees (30 seconds)

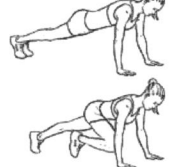

Mountain Climbers (30 seconds)

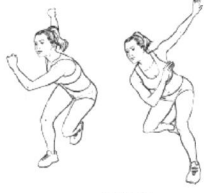

Skaters (30 seconds)

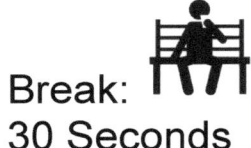

Break:
30 Seconds

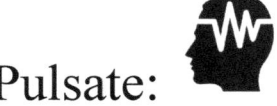

Pulsate:

go through regiment, second set (1 each) for 40 seconds (each exercise 1 time for 40 seconds) at max intensity pace focusing on maintaining target heart rate

Regiment Set 2

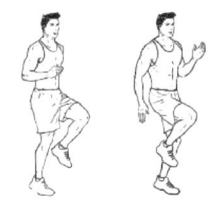

Jog in place (40 seconds)

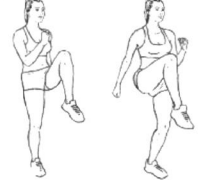

High Knees (40 seconds)

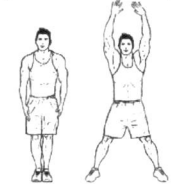

Power Jacks (40 seconds)

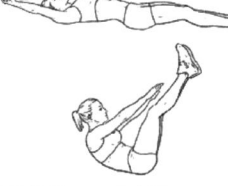

V Ups (40 seconds)

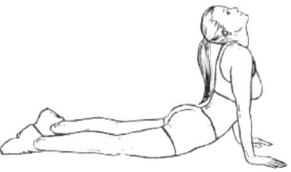

Back Extensions (40 seconds)

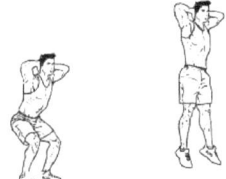

Squat Jumps (40 seconds)

Written by E Mark Pelmore

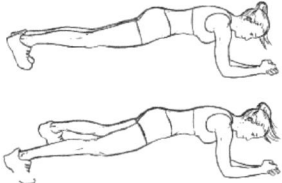

Plank Jacks (40 seconds)

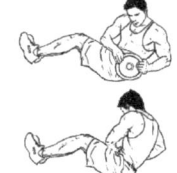

Oblique Twist (40 seconds)

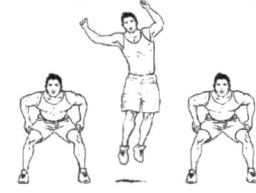

(4 = 1 ~ ←↓ →↑)

Globe Jumps (40 seconds)

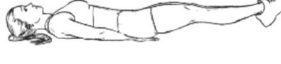

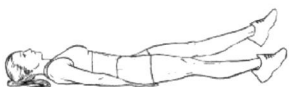

Flutter Kicks (40 seconds)

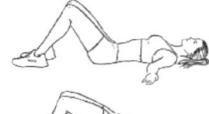

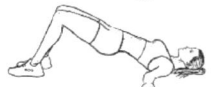

Bridge Ups (40 seconds)

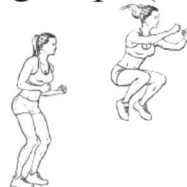

Jumping Power Knees (40 seconds)

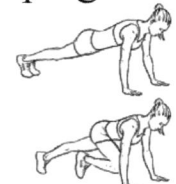

Mountain Climbers (40 seconds)

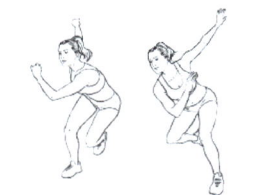

Skaters (40 seconds)

Break: 1 Minute

Cool-Down: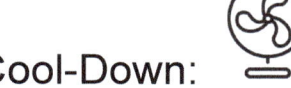

go through cool down regiment for Monday at a light pace, focusing on bringing activated muscles back to normal state and decreasing heart rate to normal levels

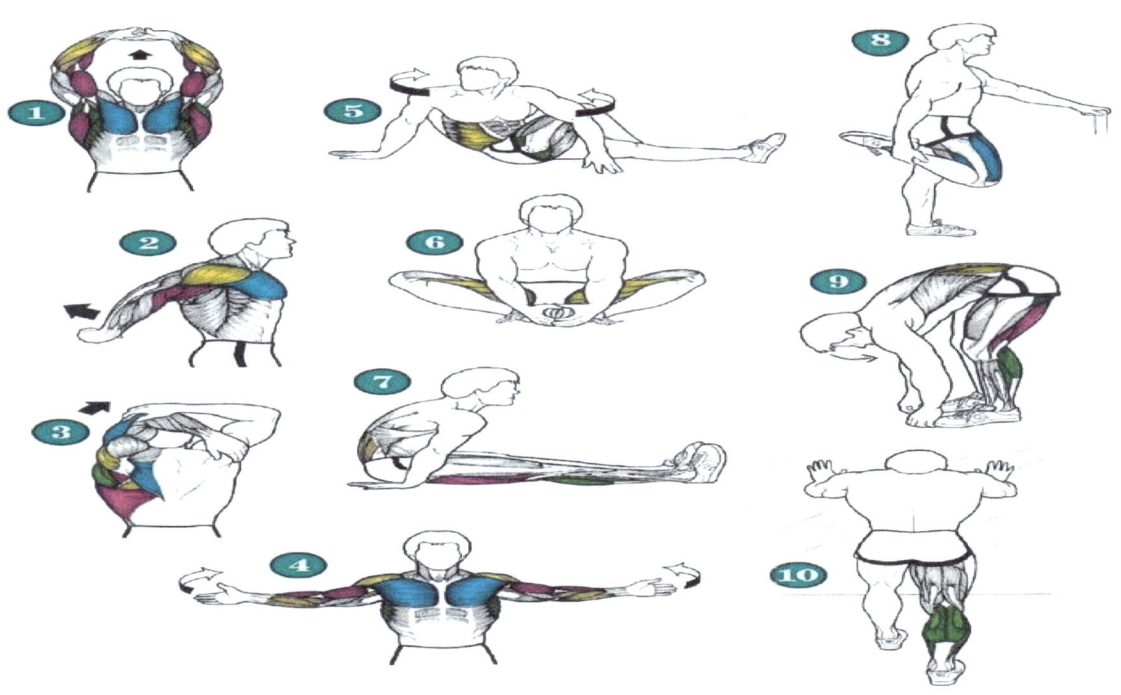

Tuesday

Nutritional Intake: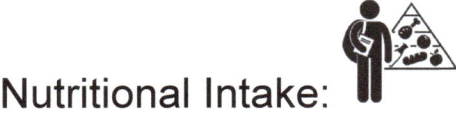

Age and gender	Estimated calories for those who do NO physically active	
	Total daily calorie needs*	Daily limit for empty calories
Girls 10-13 yrs.	1600 calories	120
Boys 10-13 yrs.	1800 calories	160
Girls 14-18 yrs.	1800 calories	160
Boys 14-18 yrs.	2200 calories	265
Females 19-30 yrs.	2000 calories	260
Males 19-30 yrs.	2400 calories	330
Females 31-50 yrs.	1800 calories	160
Males 31-50 yrs.	2200 calories	265
Females 51+ yrs.	1600 calories	120
Males 51+ yrs.	2000 calories	260

Track your Intake

Breakfast	Snack	Lunch	Snack	Dinner

Warm Up:

1 time around track at a light pace focusing on activating muscles and increasing heart rate

Stretch Out:
go through stretching regiment for Tuesday, focusing on elongating muscles

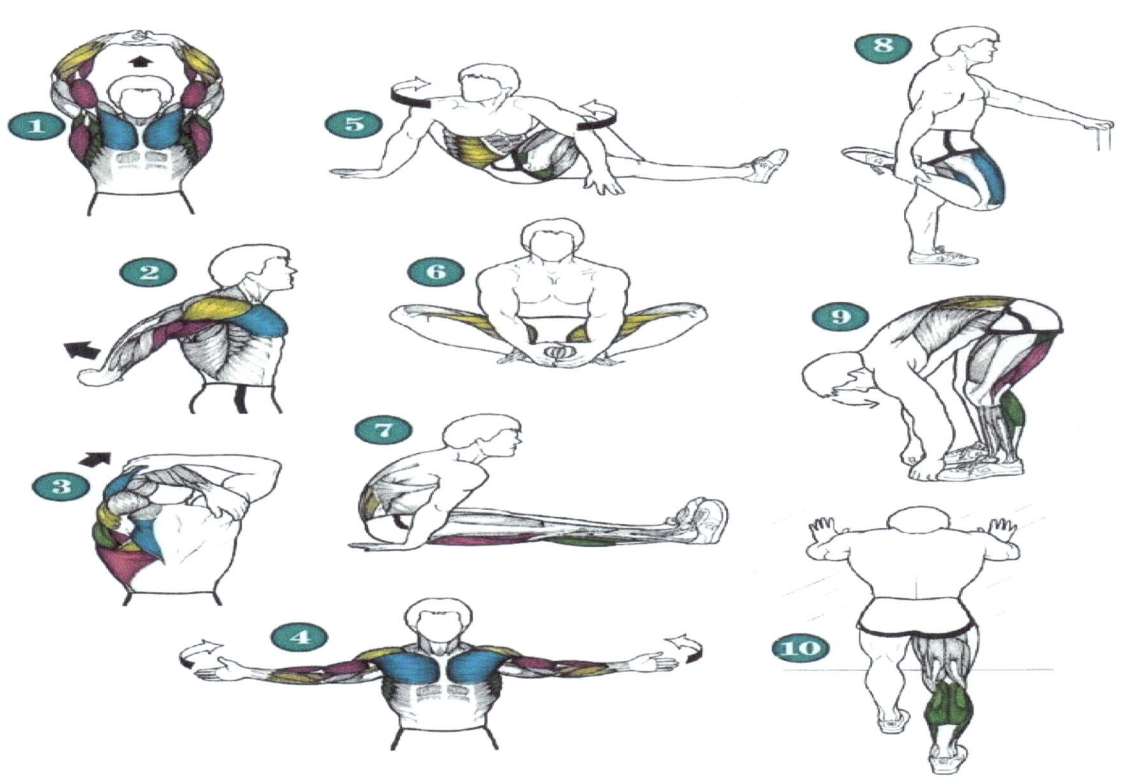

Break:
30 Seconds

Written by E Mark Pelmore

Endurance Regiment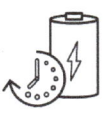

Run two (2) 400's
- At full speed

Walk a 400 between each as rest
- At brisk pace

Run five (5) 200's
- At full speed

Walk a 200 between each as rest
- At brisk pace

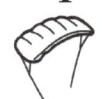

Run four (4) 60's*
- At full speed

Walk a 60 (to start) between as rest
- At brisk pace

Weight / wind-resistant if equipment available

Cool-Down:

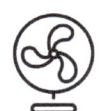

go through cool down regiment for Tuesday at a light pace, focusing on bringing activated muscles back to normal state and decreasing heart rate to normal levels

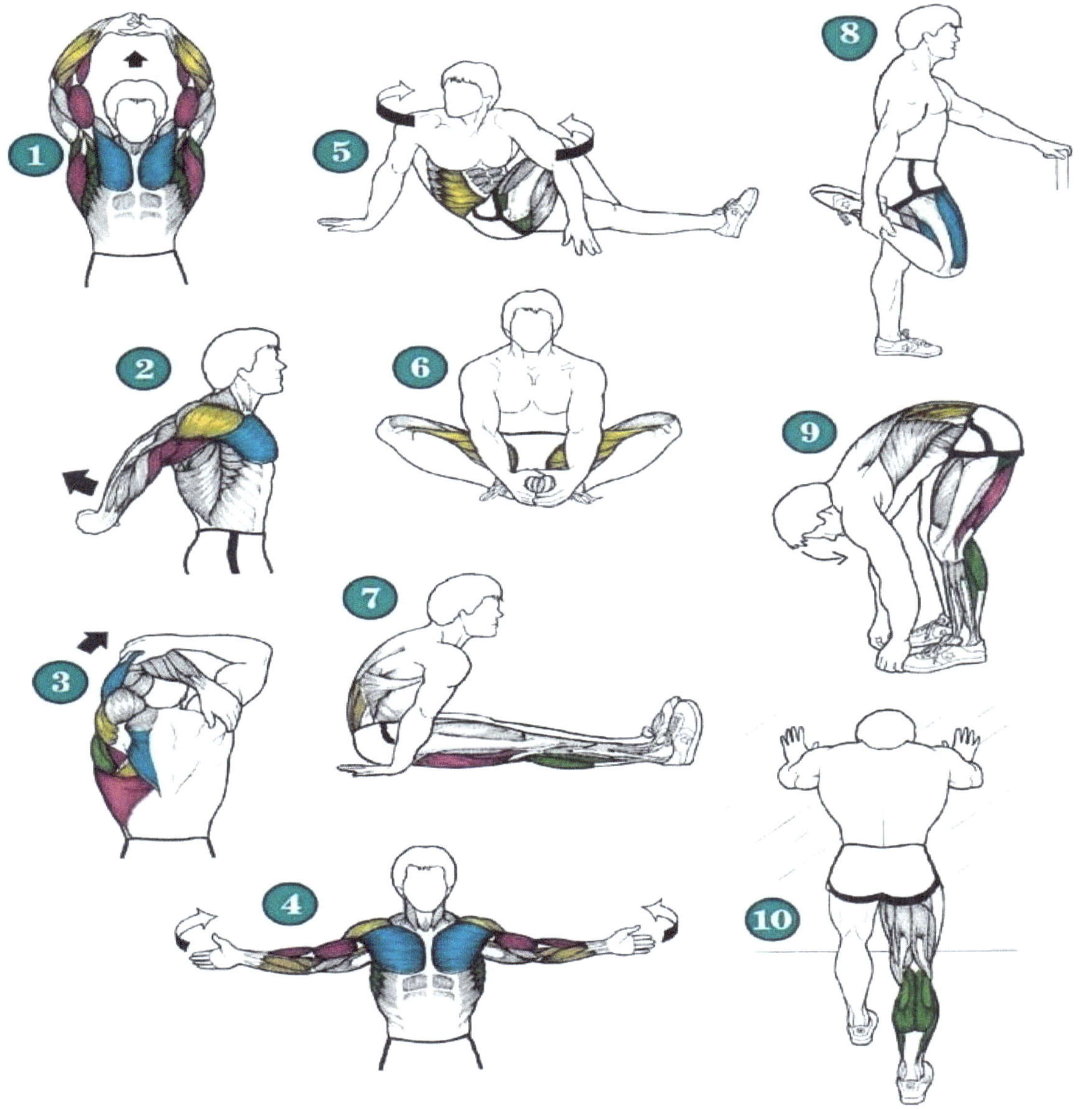

Written by E Mark Pelmore

Wednesday

Nutritional Intake:

Age and gender	Estimated calories for those who do NO physically active	
	Total daily calorie needs*	Daily limit for empty calories
Girls 10-13 yrs.	1600 calories	120
Boys 10-13 yrs.	1800 calories	160
Girls 14-18 yrs.	1800 calories	160
Boys 14-18 yrs.	2200 calories	265
Females 19-30 yrs.	2000 calories	260
Males 19-30 yrs.	2400 calories	330
Females 31-50 yrs.	1800 calories	160
Males 31-50 yrs.	2200 calories	265
Females 51+ yrs.	1600 calories	120
Males 51+ yrs.	2000 calories	260

Track your Intake

Breakfast	Snack	Lunch	Snack	Dinner

Warm Up: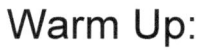

go through warm up regiment for Wednesday (each exercise 1 time for 20 seconds) at a light pace focusing on activating muscles and increasing heart rate

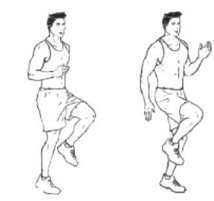

Jog in place (20 seconds)

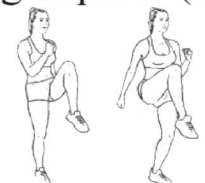

High Knees (20 seconds)

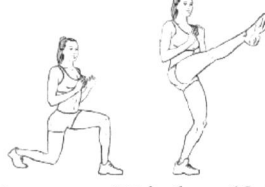

Lunge Kicks (20 seconds)

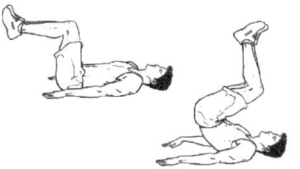

Pulse Ups (20 seconds)

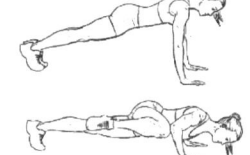

Spiderman Pushups (20 seconds)

Written by E Mark Pelmore

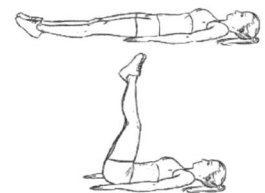

Laying Leg Raises (20 seconds)

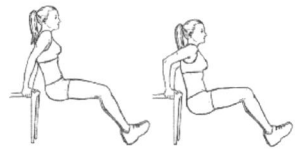

Chair Dips (20 seconds)

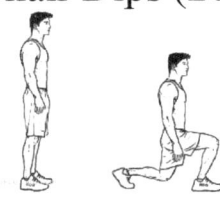

Lunges (20 seconds)

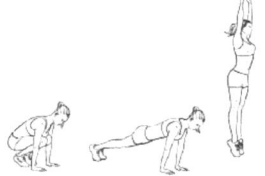

Suicide Jumps (20 seconds)

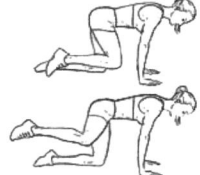

Fire Hydrants (20 seconds)

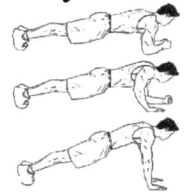

Plank to Pushup (20 seconds)

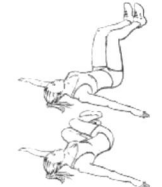

Windshield Wipers (20 seconds)

Stretch Out:

go through stretching regiment for Wednesday,
focusing on elongating muscles

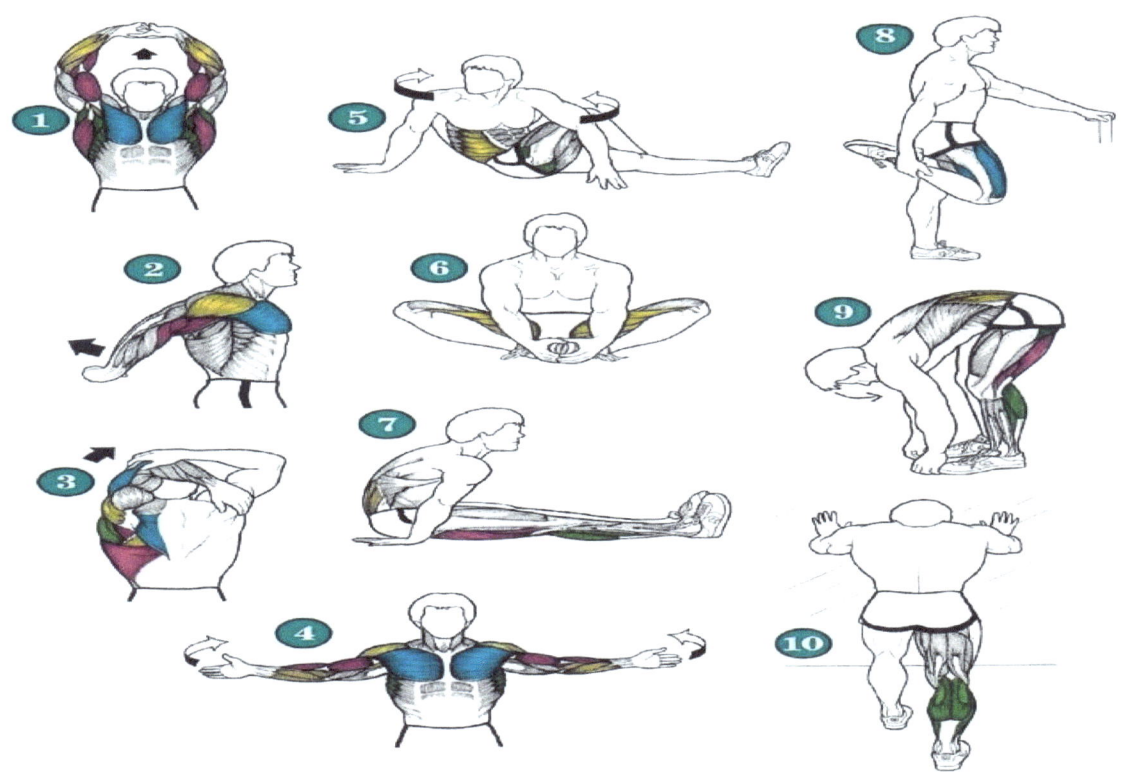

Break:

30 Seconds

Written by E Mark Pelmore

Pulsate: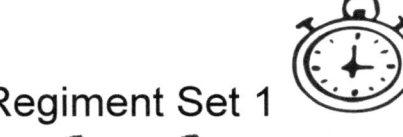

go through regiment, first set (1) time for 30 seconds
(each exercise 1 time for 30 seconds) at high intensity
pace focusing on reaching target heart rate

Regiment Set 1

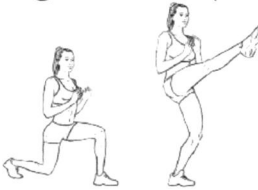

Jog in place (30 seconds)

High Knees (30 seconds)

Lunge Kicks (30 seconds)

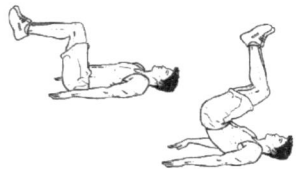

Pulse Ups (30 seconds)

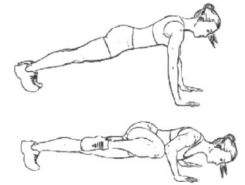

Spiderman Pushups (30 seconds)

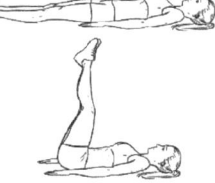

Laying Leg Raises (30 seconds)

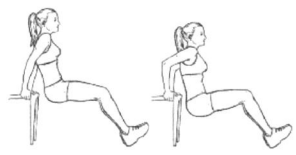

Chair Dips (30 seconds)

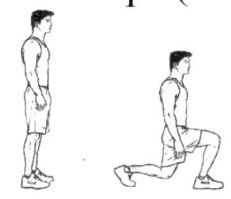

Lunges (30 seconds)

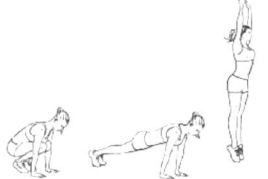

Suicide Jumps (30 seconds)

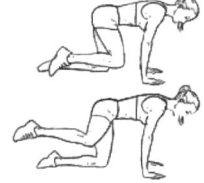

Fire Hydrants (30 seconds)

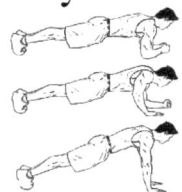

Plank to Pushup (30 seconds)

Written by E Mark Pelmore

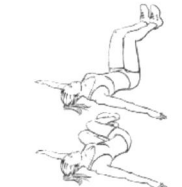

Windshield Wipers (30 seconds)

Break: 30 Seconds

Pulsate:

go through regiment, second sets (1 each) for 40 seconds (each exercise 1 time for 40 seconds) at max pace focusing on reaching target heart rate

Regiment Set 2

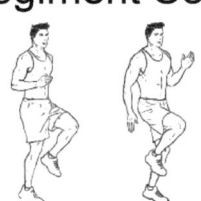

Jog in place (40 seconds)

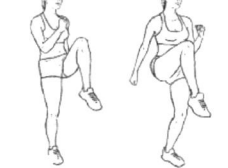

High Knees (40 seconds)

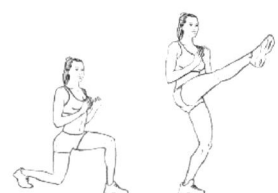

Lunge Kicks (40 seconds)

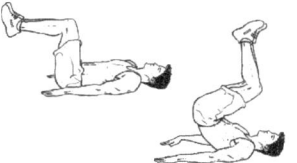

Pulse Ups (40 seconds)

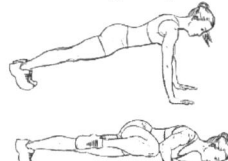

Spiderman Pushups (40 seconds)

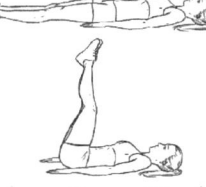

Laying Leg Raises (40 seconds)

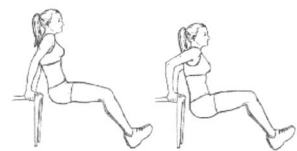

Chair Dips (40 seconds)

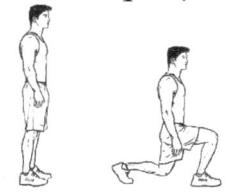

Lunges (40 seconds)

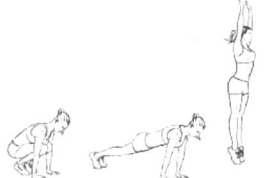

Suicide Jumps (40 seconds)

Written by E Mark Pelmore

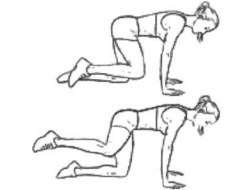

Fire Hydrants (40 seconds)

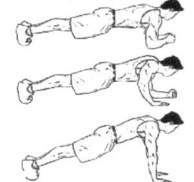

Plank to Pushup (40 seconds)

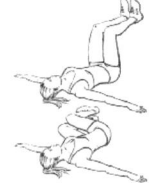

Windshield Wipers (40 seconds)

Break:
1 Minute

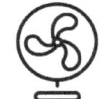

Cool-Down:

go through cool down regiment for Wednesday at a light pace, focusing on bringing activated muscles back to normal state and decreasing heart rate to normal levels

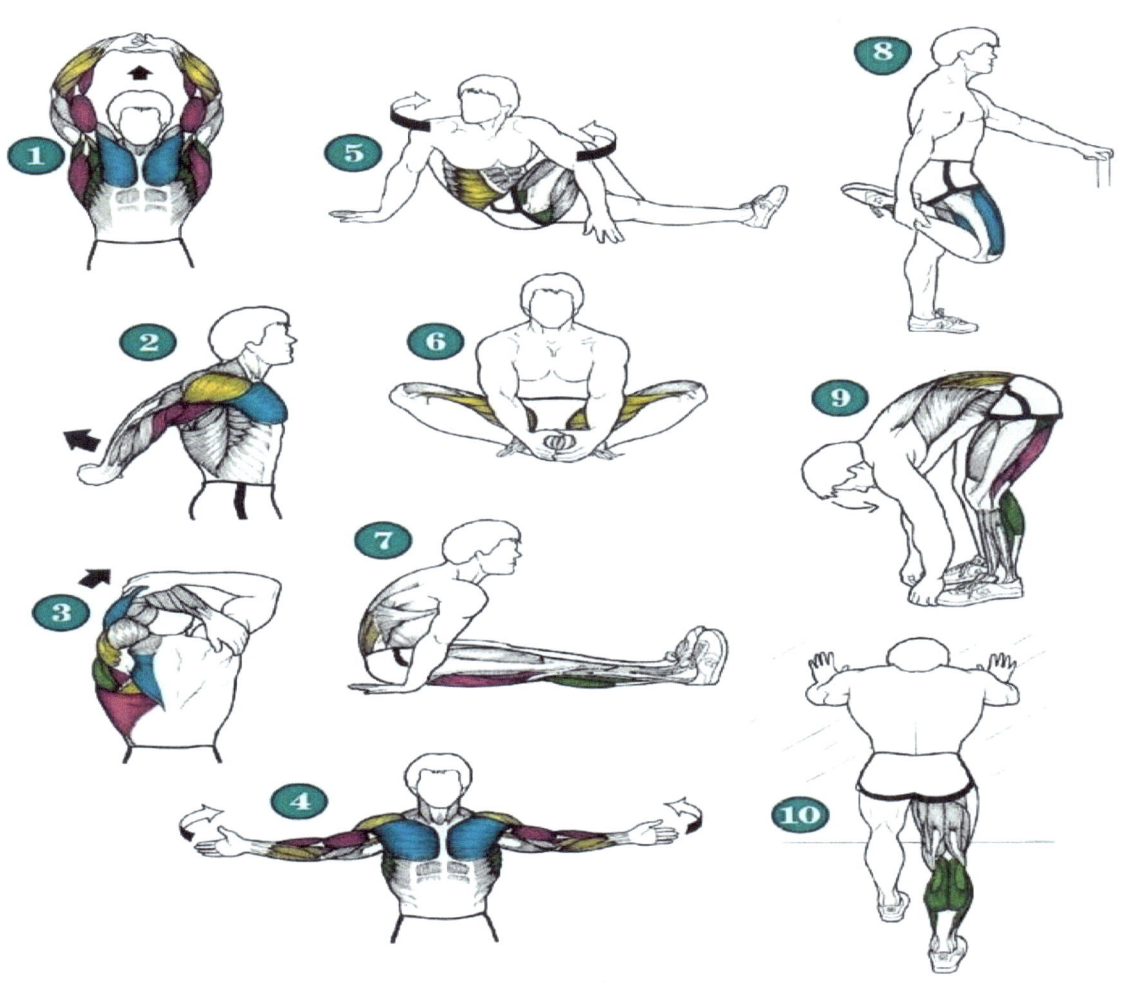

Written by E Mark Pelmore

Thursday

Nutritional Intake:

Age and gender	Estimated calories for those who do NO physically active	
	Total daily calorie needs*	Daily limit for empty calories
Girls 10-13 yrs.	1600 calories	120
Boys 10-13 yrs.	1800 calories	160
Girls 14-18 yrs.	1800 calories	160
Boys 14-18 yrs.	2200 calories	265
Females 19-30 yrs.	2000 calories	260
Males 19-30 yrs.	2400 calories	330
Females 31-50 yrs.	1800 calories	160
Males 31-50 yrs.	2200 calories	265
Females 51+ yrs.	1600 calories	120
Males 51+ yrs.	2000 calories	260

Track your Intake

Breakfast	Snack	Lunch	Snack	Dinner

Warm Up:

1 time around track at a light pace focusing on activating muscles and increasing heart rate

Stretch Out:

go through stretching regiment for Thursday, focusing on elongating muscles

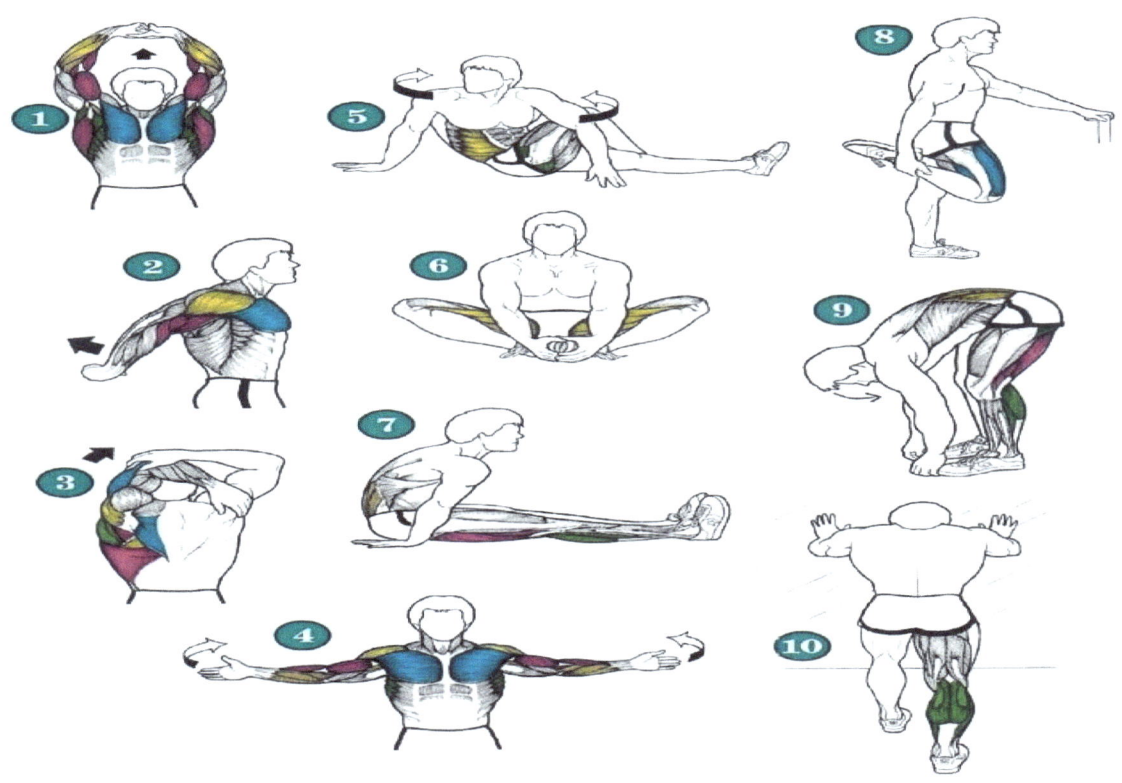

Break: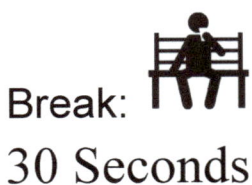

30 Seconds

Speed Regiment: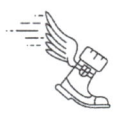

Run 5 (five) 100's
- full speed
- 40 sec rest between

Run 10 (ten) 40's
- full sprint
- 20 sec rest between

Run 20 (twenty) 10's

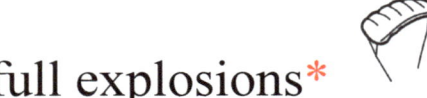

- full explosions*

* Weight / wind-resistant if equipment available

Cool-Down: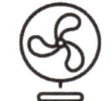

go through cool down regiment for Thursday at a light pace, focusing on bringing activated muscles back to normal state and decreasing heart rate to normal levels

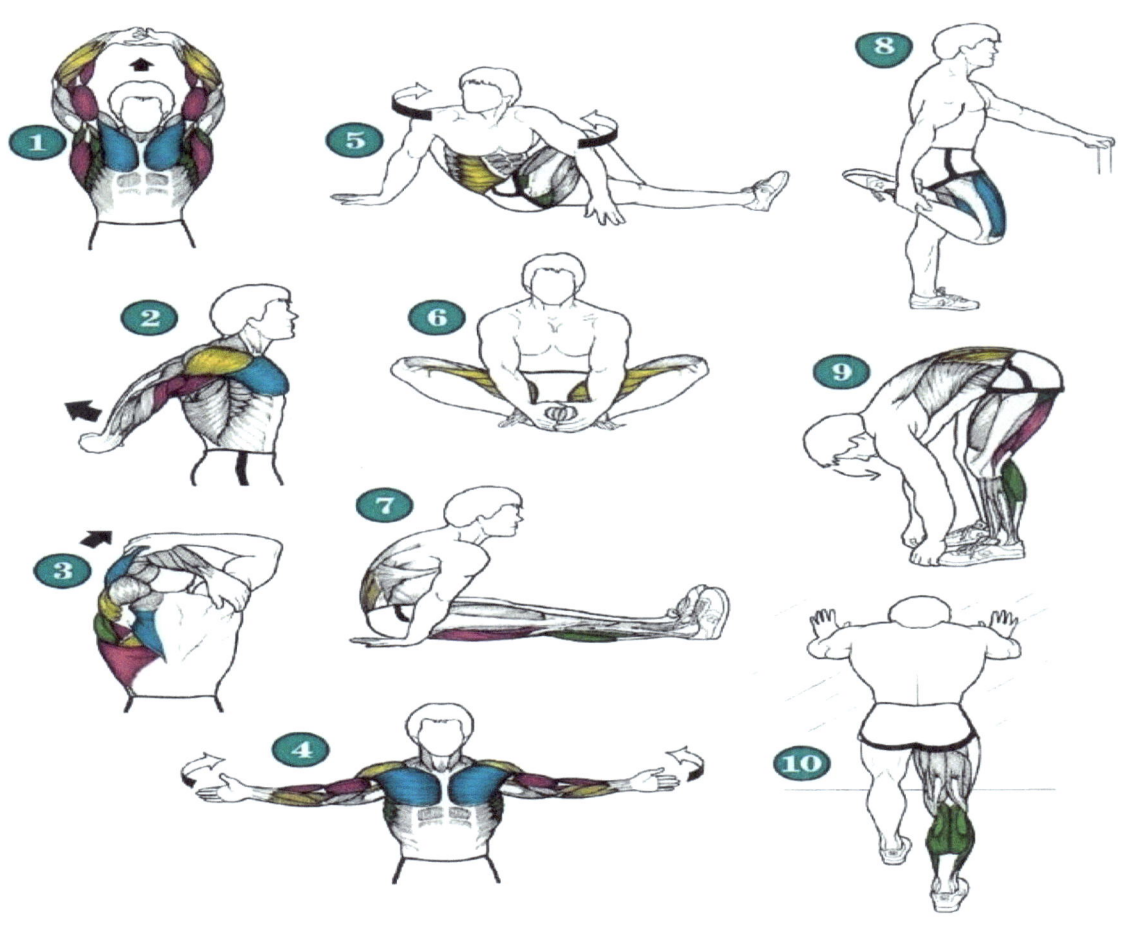

Friday

Nutritional Intake: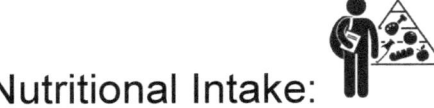

Age and gender	Estimated calories for those who do NO physically active	
	Total daily calorie needs*	Daily limit for empty calories
Girls 10-13 yrs.	1600 calories	120
Boys 10-13 yrs.	1800 calories	160
Girls 14-18 yrs.	1800 calories	160
Boys 14-18 yrs.	2200 calories	265
Females 19-30 yrs.	2000 calories	260
Males 19-30 yrs.	2400 calories	330
Females 31-50 yrs.	1800 calories	160
Males 31-50 yrs.	2200 calories	265
Females 51+ yrs.	1600 calories	120
Males 51+ yrs.	2000 calories	260

Track your Intake

Breakfast	Snack	Lunch	Snack	Dinner

Warm Up: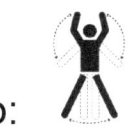

go through warm up regiment for Friday (each exercise 1 time for 20 seconds) at a light pace focusing on activating muscles and increasing heart rate

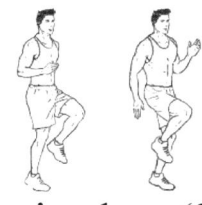

Jog in place (20 seconds)

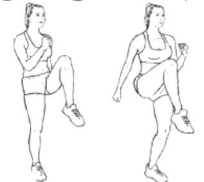

High Knees (20 seconds)

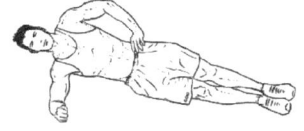

Side Plank (20 seconds)

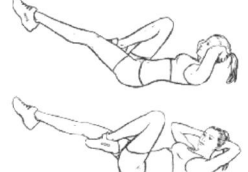

Twisting Bicycle (20 seconds)

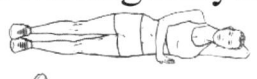

Side Leg Lifts (20 seconds)

Written by E Mark Pelmore

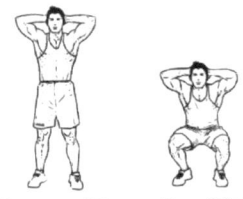

Knee Bends (20 seconds)

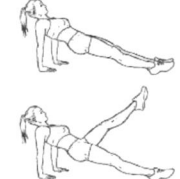

Backward Plank Kick (20 seconds)

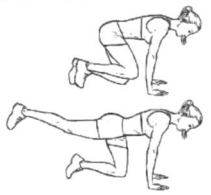

Donkey Kicks (20 seconds)

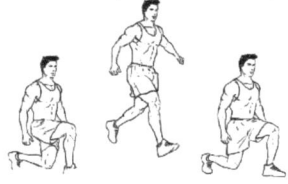

Traveling Lunge (20 seconds)

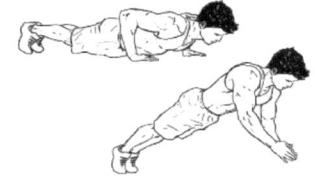

Plyo Pushups (20 seconds)

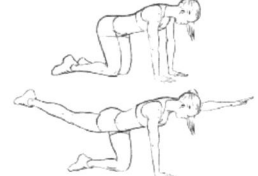

Reaching Kickbacks (20 seconds)

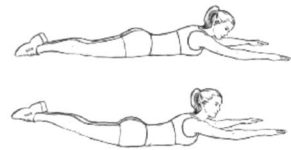

Swimmer's Stroke (20 seconds)

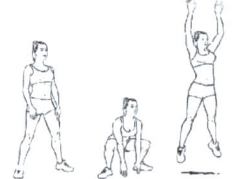

Frog Jumps (20 seconds)

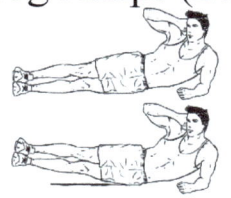

Double Jackknife (20 seconds)

Stretch Out: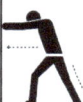

go through stretching regiment for Friday, focusing on elongating muscles

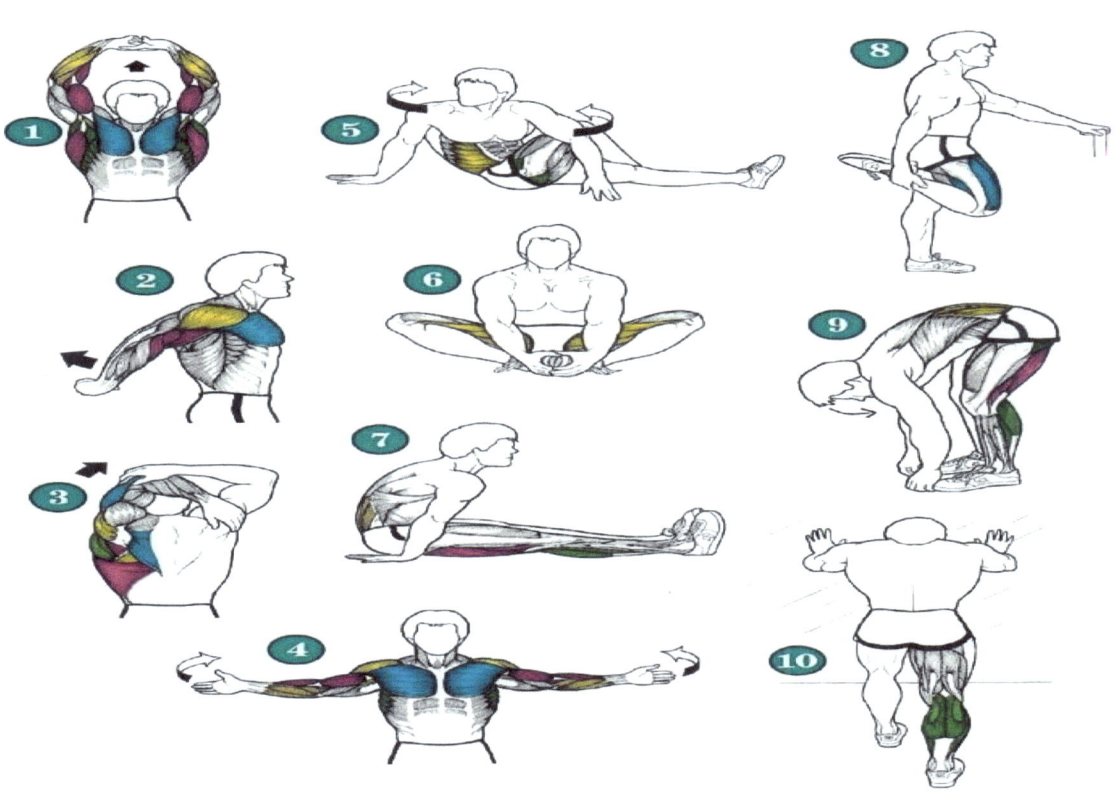

Written by E Mark Pelmore

Break: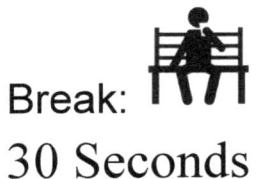

30 Seconds

Pulsate: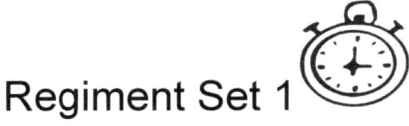

go through regiment, first set (1) time for 30 seconds
(each exercise 1 time for 30 seconds) at high intensity
pace focusing on reaching target heart rate

Regiment Set 1

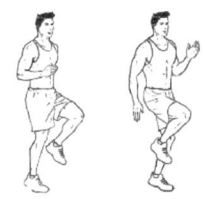

Jog in place (30 seconds)

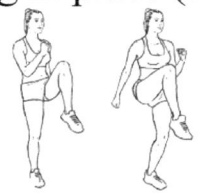

High Knees (30 seconds)

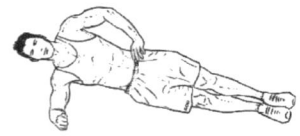

Side Plank (30 seconds)

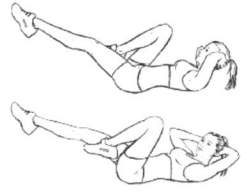

Twisting Bicycle (30 seconds)

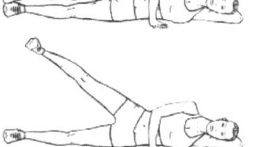

Side Leg Lifts (30 seconds)

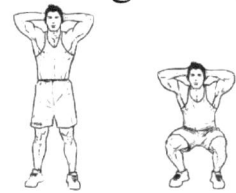

Knee Bends (30 seconds)

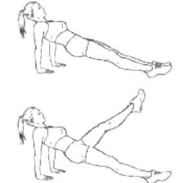

Backward Plank Kick (30 seconds)

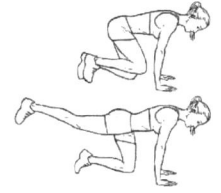

Donkey Kicks (30 seconds)

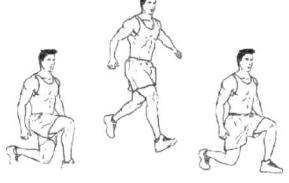

Traveling Lunge (30 seconds)

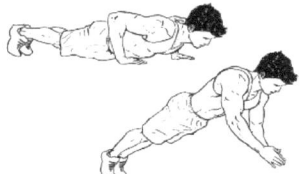

Plyo Pushups (30 seconds)

Written by E Mark Pelmore

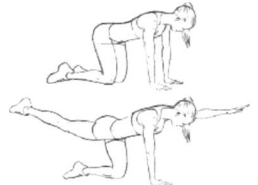

Reaching Kickbacks (30 seconds)

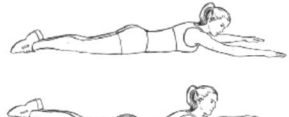

Swimmer's Stroke (30 seconds)

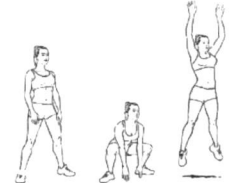

Frog Jumps (30 seconds)

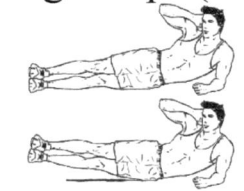

Double Jackknife (30 seconds)

Break: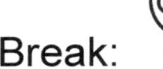
30 Seconds

Pulsate: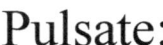
go through regiment, second set (1 each) for 40 seconds (each exercise 1 time for 40 seconds) at max pace focusing on reaching target heart rate

Regiment Set 2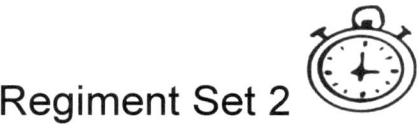

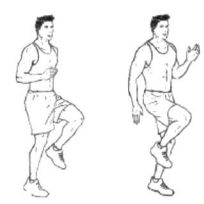

Jog in place (40 seconds)

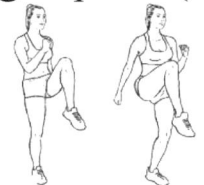

High Knees (40 seconds)

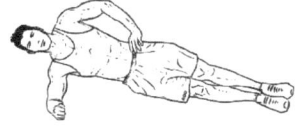

Side Plank (40 seconds)

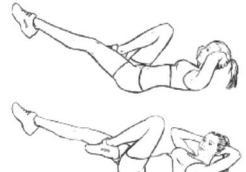

Twisting Bicycle (40 seconds)

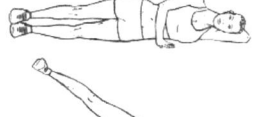

Side Leg Lifts (40 seconds)

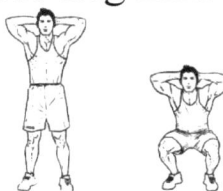

Knee Bends (40 seconds)

Written by E Mark Pelmore

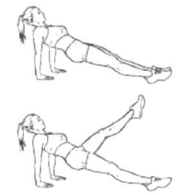

Backward Plank Kick (40 seconds)

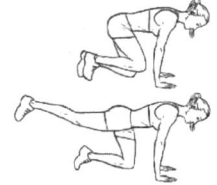

Donkey Kicks (40 seconds)

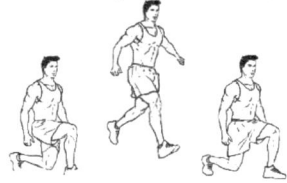

Traveling Lunge (40 seconds)

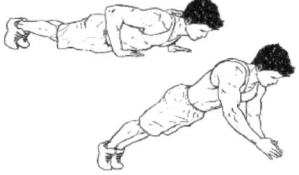

Plyo Pushups (40 seconds)

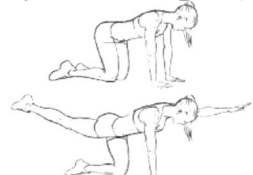

Reaching Kickbacks (40 seconds)

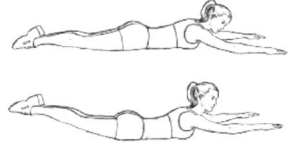

Swimmer's Stroke (40 seconds)

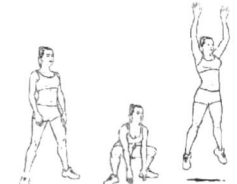

Frog Jumps (40 seconds)

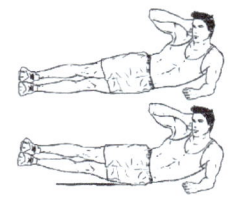

Double Jackknife (40 seconds)

Break: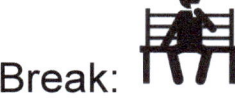

1 Minute

Cool-Down: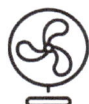

go through cool down regiment for Friday at a light pace focusing on bringing activated muscles back to normal state and decreasing heart rate to normal levels

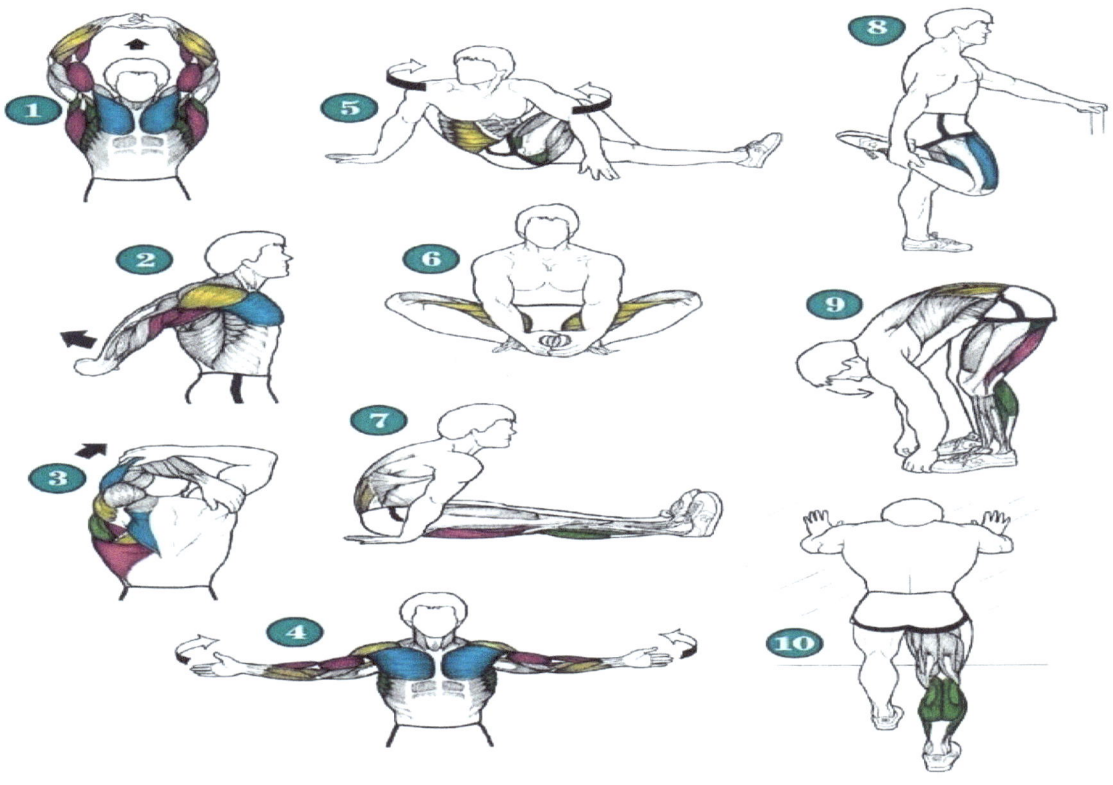

Saturday

Nutritional Intake: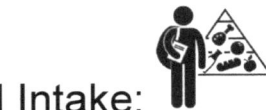

Age and gender	Estimated calories for those who do NO physically active	
	Total daily calorie needs*	Daily limit for empty calories
Girls 10-13 yrs.	1600 calories	120
Boys 10-13 yrs.	1800 calories	160
Girls 14-18 yrs.	1800 calories	160
Boys 14-18 yrs.	2200 calories	265
Females 19-30 yrs.	2000 calories	260
Males 19-30 yrs.	2400 calories	330
Females 31-50 yrs.	1800 calories	160
Males 31-50 yrs.	2200 calories	265
Females 51+ yrs.	1600 calories	120
Males 51+ yrs.	2000 calories	260

Track your Intake

Breakfast	Snack	Lunch	Snack	Dinner

Warm Up: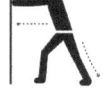

As appropriate for the cardio selection

Stretch Out: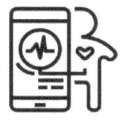

as instructed before the cardio selection

Cardio Regiment:

(Choose 1 cardio exercise)
Lasting 30 - 40 min per session:

 Water Aerobics

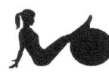 Dance Experience

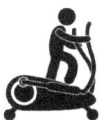 Pilates

  Stationary Machine

  Yoga

Zumba

Written by E Mark Pelmore

Pulsate: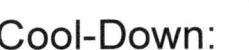

go through the Cardio selection at your max pace focusing on reaching target heart rate

Cool-Down:

Go through cool down as instructed by Cardio selection

Alternative Selections

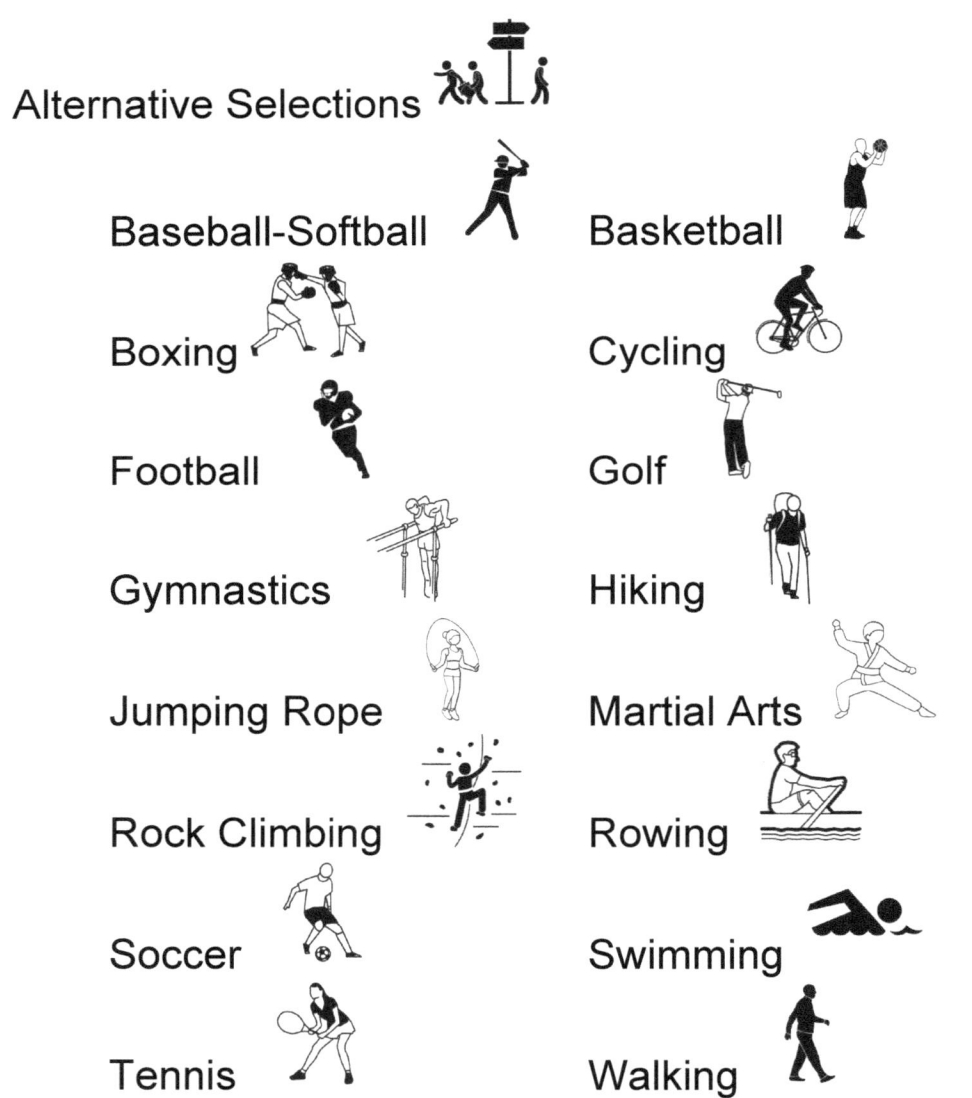

Baseball-Softball

Basketball

Boxing

Cycling

Football

Golf

Gymnastics

Hiking

Jumping Rope

Martial Arts

Rock Climbing

Rowing

Soccer

Swimming

Tennis

Walking